Bella's Heart Surgery Story

VICTORIA LOVE

AuthorHouse™
1663 Liberty Drive
Bloomington, IN 47403
www.authorhouse.com
Phone: 1 (833) 262-8899

This book is printed on acid-free paper.

ISBN: 978-1-6655-0418-8 (sc)
ISBN: 978-1-6655-0419-5 (e)

Library of Congress Control Number: 2020920106

Print information available on the last page.

Published by AuthorHouse 10/15/2020

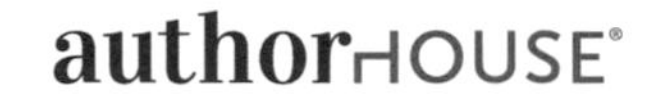

BELLA'S HEART SURGERY STORY

On December 14, 2019 around 9:00 p.m., mommy was at Uncle Jeff's house socializing with family and his county co-workers for his annual Holiday party. Your Uncle Jeff was the Chairman of Clayton County, Georgia at the time. While sitting at the table and eating with other family members, mommy started having severe squeezing pains in her tummy. I did not think they were contractions, but maybe Braxton Hicks, which is pain pregnant women get before they have actual real contractions which allow all mommies to know their bundle of joy is on the way. After a few of those your cousin Jami and Aunt Deborah kept saying, "Victoria I believe you are having contractions. Aunt Deborah started timing the contractions and told me that when the pain becomes five minutes apart, I need to call the doctor or go to the hospital." You had a hard head mom at that time, so I just went home and prepared for work for the next morning. Mommy was a bartender and manager at a Sushi restaurant at the time, as well as a special needs teacher.

That next morning was Sunday December 15, 2019, as soon as I got to work my pains grew worst. I called your Aunt Jan to see if she thought they were labor pains or Braxton Hicks. Aunt Jan said, "Victoria you need to leave work! Do not drive home, me, and Uncle Aundre will come get you and drive your car home. It sounds like you are having contractions. Are you timing them?" Again, you had a hard head mother and I drove home anyways. The second I got on the interstate I realized I should have listened to Aunt Jan. But mommy made it home safe about 5:00 p.m. I went in the house, ate, and fell asleep until 11:00 p.m.

I slept with your Aunt Tracei'a that night and woke her up saying, "Sis, get up I think I need to go to the hospital now." No, my water did not break but the pains grew worst. It felt like someone was twisting muscles in my stomach not bad cramps like I was told contractions would feel like. That is when I learned no women delivery pains are the same.

When I checked into the hospital at 12:37 a.m. on December 16, 2019, the nurse said, "My goodness we have another baby possibly being delivered today. You are the 4th pregnant women to check in, in the last 24 minutes." Once I was checked in and into a room, the nurse checked my cervices to see how far I had dilated. I had only dilated 1 centimeter, which was not good. A baby comes at 10 centimeters. I was sure they were getting ready to send me home. The doctor came in and checked me 10 minutes later, and at that time I had dilated 4 centimeters.

THE BABY IS COMING!!! THE BABY IS COMING!!! THE BABY IS COMING!!!

Dr. Taylor tells the nurse to move me across the hall to the actual delivery room. It was a nice room. Dr. Taylor gave me some medicine that seemed like it only lasted five minutes. Mommy was a clown. Bella, I kept trying to stand up on the table and I kept telling the doctor "I can't do it. The baby is squeezing my muscles in my stomach." Your granny and auntie just sat staring at me. The doctor is yelling, "No Victoria you cannot do that sit down. I will give you something to curve the pain." It helped mommy for a short period of time. Minutes after that the nurse gave me an Epidural, that is a shot they put in mommy spine area in her back. Most women get this shot at the time of delivery to numb your body so you can tolerate the pain. I did not see the actual needle, but Aunt Tracei'a says it was a large needle that the nurse stuck me with three times. I will say it helped a lot and it was worth having at the time. I did not feel the needle when they put it in my back. I only felt a little pinch. Once the epidural was administered, I was able to sit back and relax for a few minutes before Dr. Taylor came back in the room walking back and forth staring at mommy. I hear him mumbling amongst the other nurses and immediately I knew something was wrong. He left out the room and came back a second time with a paper for me to sign. Telling me, "can you sign this paper just in case we need to do a C-section, it states that nothing is wrong, but we may have to prepare for it just in case." He then asked, "When did you go into labor?" I really did not know. I realized I may have been in labor when Jami and Aunt Deborah told me I was. That meant I went into labor two days ago but was naïve about what was happening, believing the pains would have been worse than what they were. I told him "two days ago." He looks at me and said, "TWO DAYS AGO!!! WHY ARE YOU JUST COMING IN?!! He looks at Aunt Tracei'a and questions her. She was like, "I didn't know." That is your Aunt Tracei'a favorite phase to say when she is under pressure. He leaves the room again and comes back five minutes later saying they would have to do an emergency C-section. I was happy about having the C-section, only because I honestly did not want to push and was scared to have a vaginal birth. What worried me was I knew something could have been wrong with you now.

Dr. Taylor said, "Victoria, listen to me everything is going to be okay. Remember when I told you we may have to do a C-section? Well we need to do one and we need to do it NOW. You are continuing to dilate, and this baby has not dropped at all. You will be in labor for days at this point. Your contractions are extremely strong and every time you have a contraction this baby heart rate is dropping." I looked at the clock and it is exactly 4:11 a.m. The nurses picked me up and put me on another bed and begin to roll me to the surgery table. I see another nurse handing granny some type of gown to put on so she can come with me to the operating room. Aunt Tracei'a was not able to come back because only one person was allowed in the operating room with me. So, Aunt Tracei'a waited in the waiting room. Once I went to the surgery room, I could feel Dr. Taylor rubbing something on my stomach then asking me, "Can you feel me poking you?" I replied no. Not realizing he had already started the procedure, cutting mommy open. No, I could not see anything because they had me strapped to a cold table and a large blue tarp blocking me from seeing anything. I was mad at Granny I could not understand what was taking her so long to come with me when she was right across the hall. When granny finally came in, Dr. Taylor was pulling you out. Right after he pulled you out your grandma was sitting beside me. I yelled Doctor, "I have to vomit" he yelled back "hold your head to the side". A nurse in the room gave granny a cup to hold over my mouth. I guess she was too excited she held the cup over my nose instead of my mouth. Not only could I not breathe but I vomit on myself and the floor. Mommy was so mad. I had to lay there with vomit on me until the operation was over. The second you came out Dr. Taylor yells, "what is the time." Someone yells back 4:35 a.m. I said to myself, jeez it took less than 20 mins and thought to myself that was great.

Then I hear Dr. Taylor say, "Why is this baby breathing so fast? She is so small. What is her weight?" A nurse yells back she is 4.9 pounds. I hear Dr. Taylor say, "something is wrong. This baby is too small, how many weeks is she?" At this point I knew something was wrong but was still happy you were alive. I could not hold you because I was still tied to the table getting my stomach stitched up. Granny walked you over to me holding you so I could see you. You winked your right eye at me, and I winked back. You had a cry so light we barley heard you crying. They cleaned you up and took you straight to the NICU (Neonatal Intensive Care Unit).

LIFE IN THE NICU

Mommy was rolled back to her room after surgery at 7:36 a.m. When I got back to the room Aunt Tracei'a was there and two hours later granny came back to the room. While we talked for a few minutes your grandfather in Texas called to tell us your Uncle Prentiss had passed. Mommy was such a mess to hear this and I did not have my baby with me either. My day was already going bad. Granny went back to the NICU with the nurse and stayed with you till Aunt Tracei'a and I came down to the NICU around 12:00 p.m. to see you. I had to come in a wheelchair. When I came to the NICU they had you in an oxygen tent, not an incubator or ventilator but an oxygen tent machine to help with your breathing.

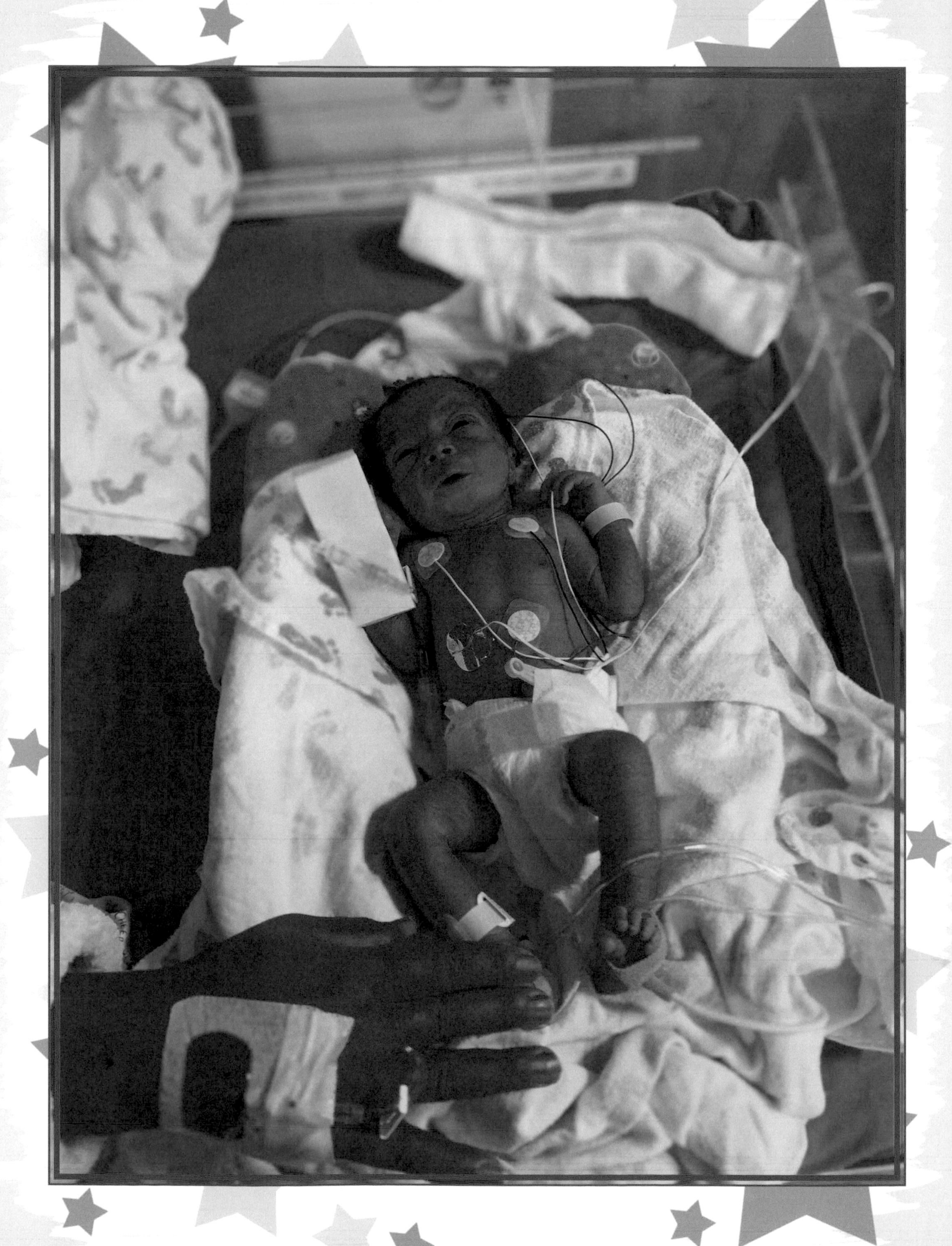

Mommy came two more times that day to see you before actually being able to get a little sleep. The next day, granny and Aunt Tracei'a, your cousin and godmother Kenisha came and stayed with mommy for two days at the hospital. While Kenisha and I were in mommy's room talking and laughing Dr. Stone the Neonatal doctor came in with his 'NO HAVING BED SIDE MANNER SLEF' and says, "Hello are you Bella's mom? Before I could answer he says, "Well I am going to tell you just like this, she ain't going home no time soon. We are running a few tests on her and it appears she has heart failure." And he walked out the room. Kenisha and I looked at each other in shock, like he is a rude joker. I had tears in my eyes and tried to get up saying to Kenisha, "this is not the real doctor" she says, "hold on let's go check on Bella, let me grab a wheelchair for you." We both were quiet, it seemed like the longest walk and elevator ride ever to get to you. When I saw you, there were two open cuts on both sides of your neck. Mommy questioned about why the cuts were there and that opened a can of worms. I thought it came from the c-section, but Dr. Stone said it was everything but anything positive (which did not make sense). When mommy came back down to visit you, I had to wear a mask, gown and gloves as if I was getting ready to perform a surgery. Dr. Stone thought you had a virus because of the neck bruises and wanted everyone that came in your presence to be cautious and wear this attire. Everything came back negative. Mommy believe the marks on your neck came from the c-section procedure. When you get older you will still see the marks on your neck, they never went away. After one month of sitting in the NICU, Dr. Stone explained you had two holes in your heart one was a Patent Ductus Arteriosus (PDA) and the other was called Ventricular Septal Defect (VSD). PDA is a persistent opening between the two major blood vessels leading from the heart. Usually everyone is born with an open PDA, but it is supposed to close within 24 hours. Your PDA hole never closed. A (**VSD**) is a hole in the wall separating the two lower chambers of the heart.

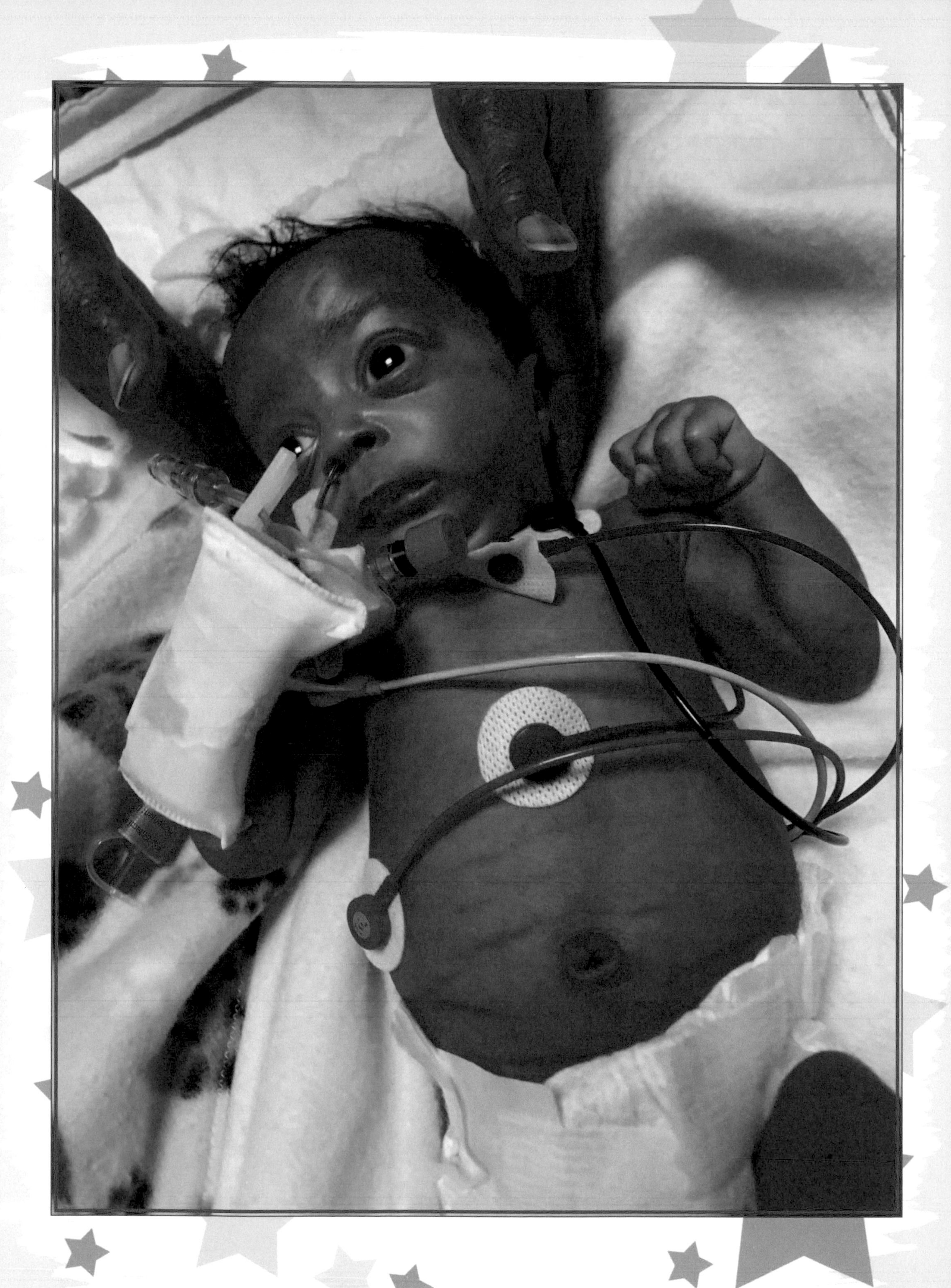

Two months later, on January 22, 2020 when I came to the hospital to check on you Dr. Stone says they are going to let you come home. Yes, I was a little nervous about it because I was thinking if her PDA and VSD holes are still open she will not live long like this. The next day Dr. Stone calls with a cardiologist on the phone, “Ms. Love this is Dr. Stone I have a cardiologist with me. Now you can take her home today or she can be transferred to the other hospital it is up to you. I don’t know what they will do different than what our hospital has done.” Then the cardiologist got on the phone saying, “Hello Ms. Love, I am a cardiologist from the other hospital, I am the one making recommendation that Bella gets transferred. She is in NO condition to go home.” I tell her Thank you, yes, I want her transferred. The cardiologist says “Great I will try and have her moved today if there is a bed available at the other hospital. If not, today she will be moved tomorrow.” I was so happy to hear this and knew it was God moving you because the hospital you were at now was not able to help you it had already been two months and there was no progress. You did need to be at a children’s hospital that specialized with children and hearts.

NEW HOSPITAL NEW BEGINNING NEW HOSPITAL

On February 24, 2020, mommy got up early to be with you as they prepared for you to depart from your current hospital to your new beginnings. At 3:00 p.m. a neonatal ambulance came to pick you up to transfer you to a Children's hospital in Atlanta, Georgia. As we left the nurses at the hospital who took great care of you for the last two months cried as the first responders loaded you up to leave. It was a sad moment for mommy too. I did not know what to except next, but I knew God was in control. I tried hard not to worry but that is easier said than done.

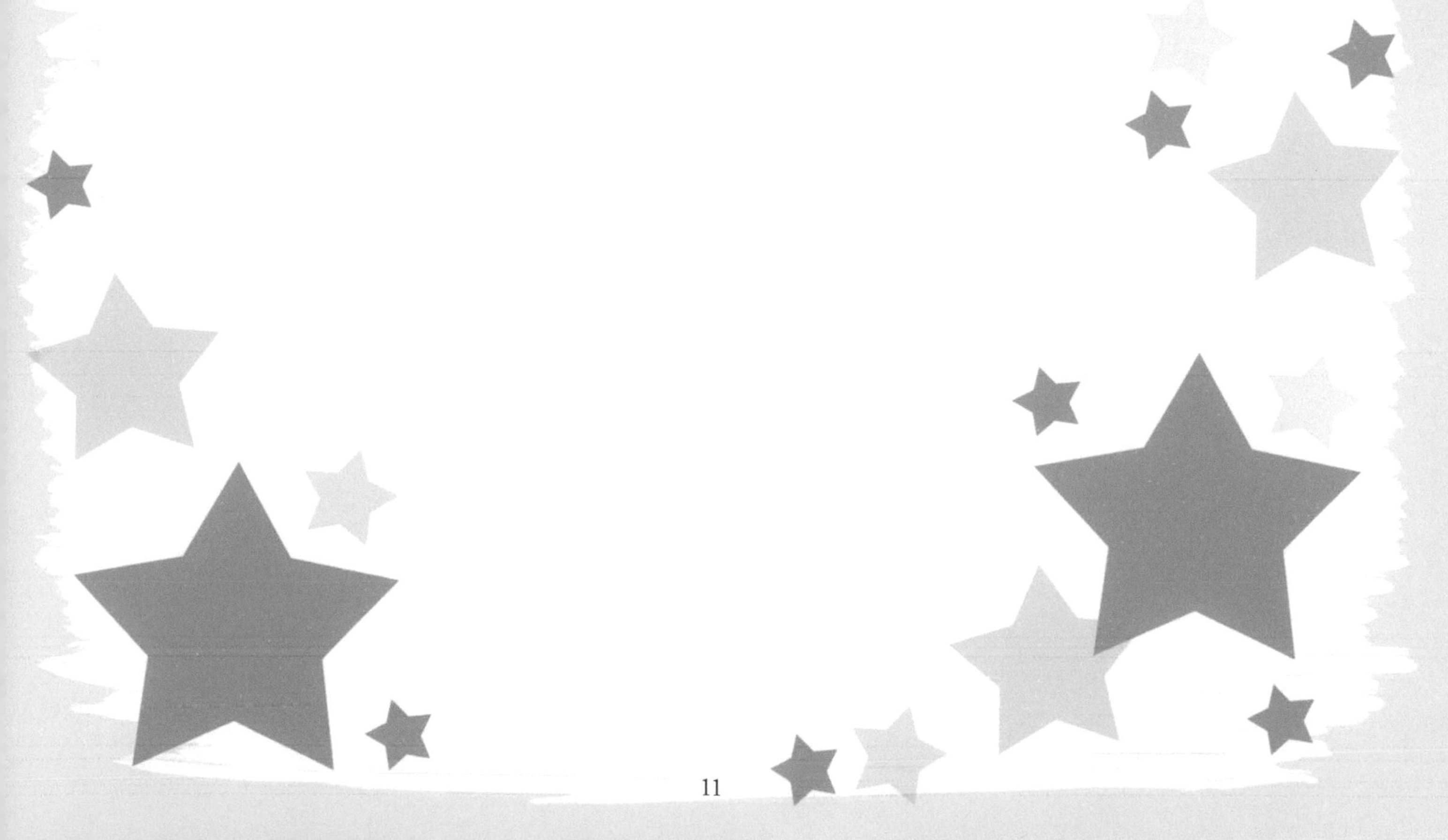

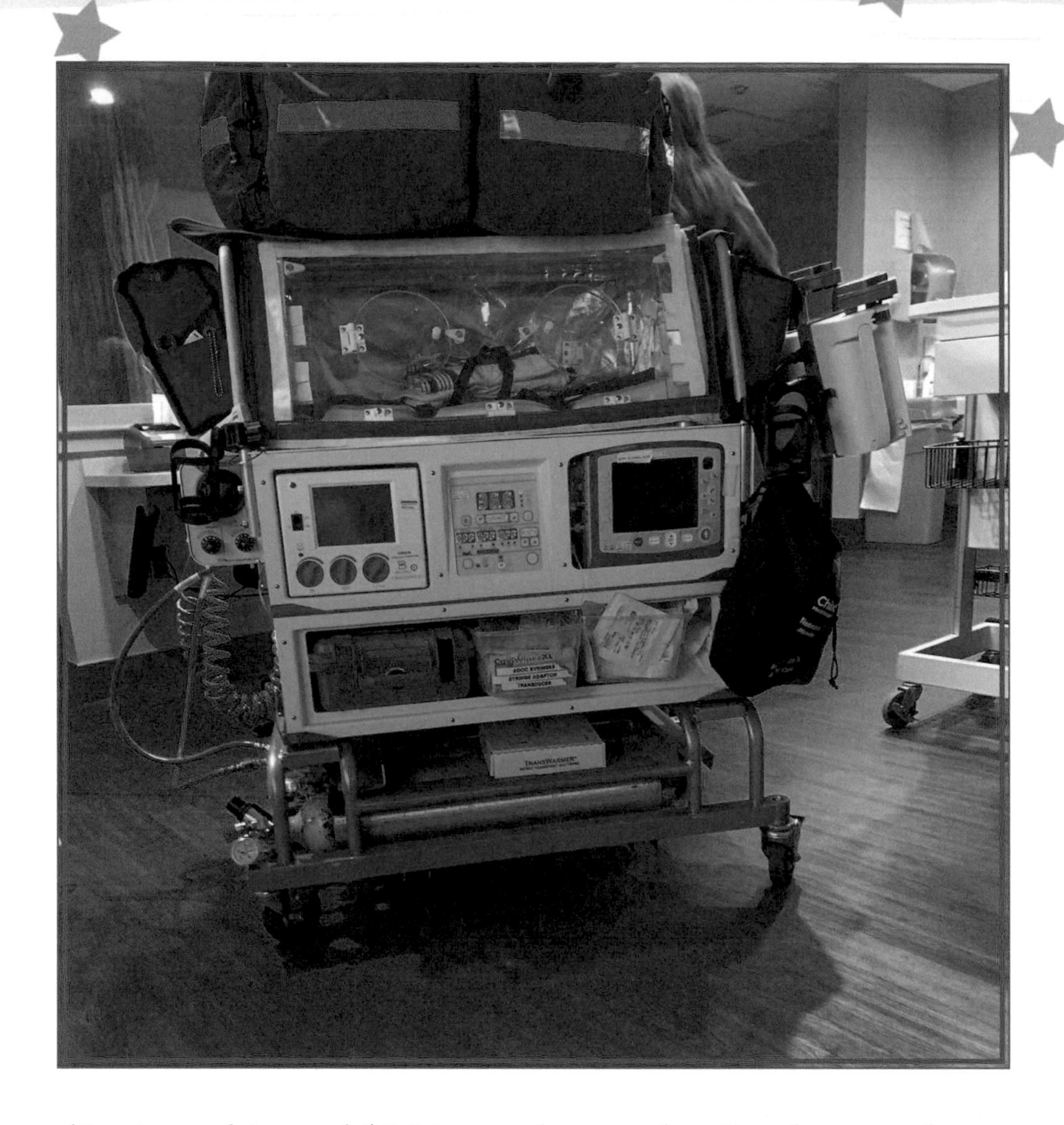

It was a 45-minute drive and $5.00 to park every day. But that was okay, you were my baby and gas prices were only $2.37 at the time. It took mommy $24.00 to fill her Mini Cooper Countryman up. The nurses and doctors at the children's hospital were beyond nice and loving people. They were more like flower children, nice and happy people. It only took them four days to confirm you did have heart failure and a week more to decide to have heart surgery or to place a stent called a catheter, which they would have stuck in the vein of your thigh that goes up to your heart.

On Monday February 3, 2020, around 10:00 a.m., mommy was at work when a nurse called and said, "Ms. Love, Bella will be having heart surgery tomorrow morning." I stood outside the school gym in shock, scared and crying. I then went back to my class, having a hard time trying to handle the thought of you having heart surgery due to fear that something could happen to you. I was thinking today could be the last day I hold or kiss my baby alive. When I went back to my classroom, one of the custodians I was friends with was in the room and talked to me about what was going on. He told me to make sure I asked the doctor questions such as, “How long will the surgery take? Will she have to have any more surgeries after this? How long will the healing process take?” That is exactly what I asked as soon as I spoke with the doctor later that day. When I left work, I immediately called my other job at the Sushi Bar to let them know I was not coming in so I could stay with you the whole night before your surgery in the morning.

At 5:30 am on February 4, 2020, an hour before your original scheduled surgery time, they canceled it and rescheduled for the next morning. There was another baby who had to have emergency surgery, so you were bumped that day. Mommy, Granny and Aunt Tracei’a missed work again on Wednesday to be with you for surgery and at 6:00 a.m. a nurse comes in saying you were bumped again because of another baby who was more important than you. I honestly do not think she meant it the way she said it, but it broke my heart and made me feel like my baby heart was not as important as the other babies. Day 3, it is Thursday and they bump you again and I snapped.

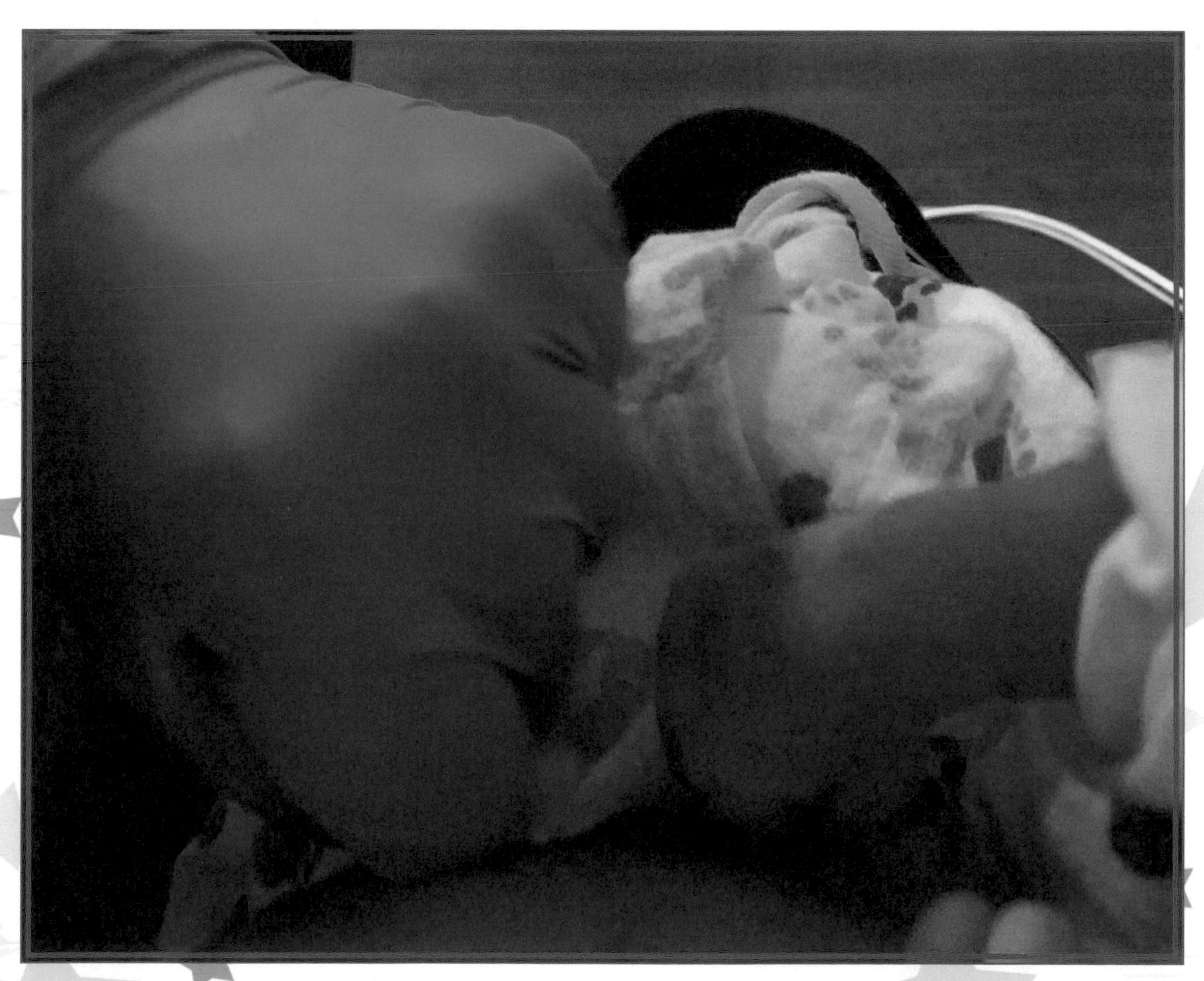

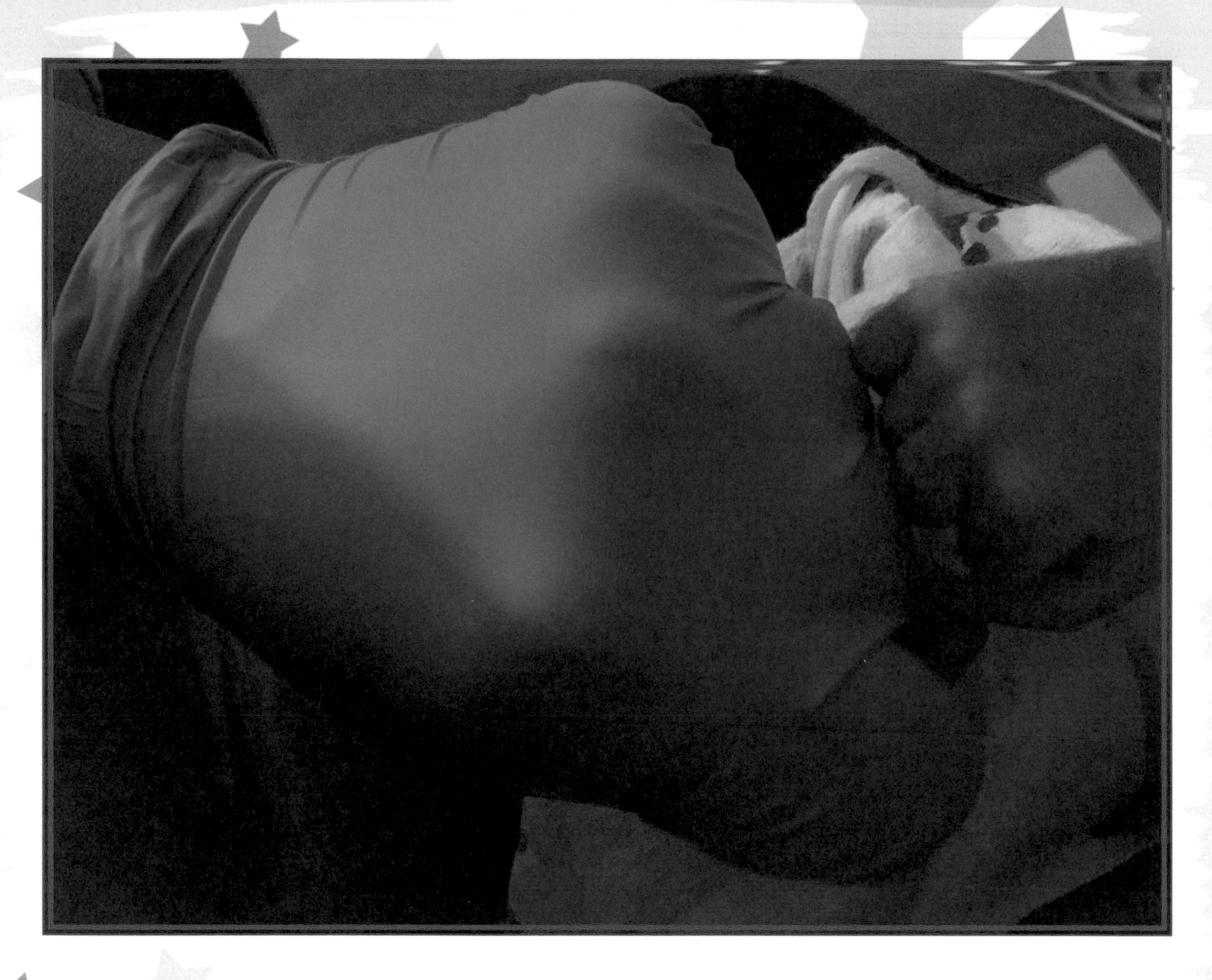

Finally, your heart surgery was performed on Friday February 7, 2020 around 9:00 a.m. Mommy was not there for the actual surgery because I was not sure the actual surgery would happen due to the frequent delays. Honestly, mommy was sort of embarrassed for snapping off at the nurses and doctors after they delayed your surgery the third time. That played a big part of why I did not make it on time for the surgery, besides the fact mommy worked about 45 minutes from the hospital. Your Aunt Jan and Aunt Deborah told me to walk in that hospital and hold my head high and act like nothing ever happen about me snapping off. As soon as I arrived at the hospital at 11:30 a.m. that is exactly what I did. I walked in like a sane normal mommy and your surgery was already done and you were in ICU sleeping the anesthesia off.

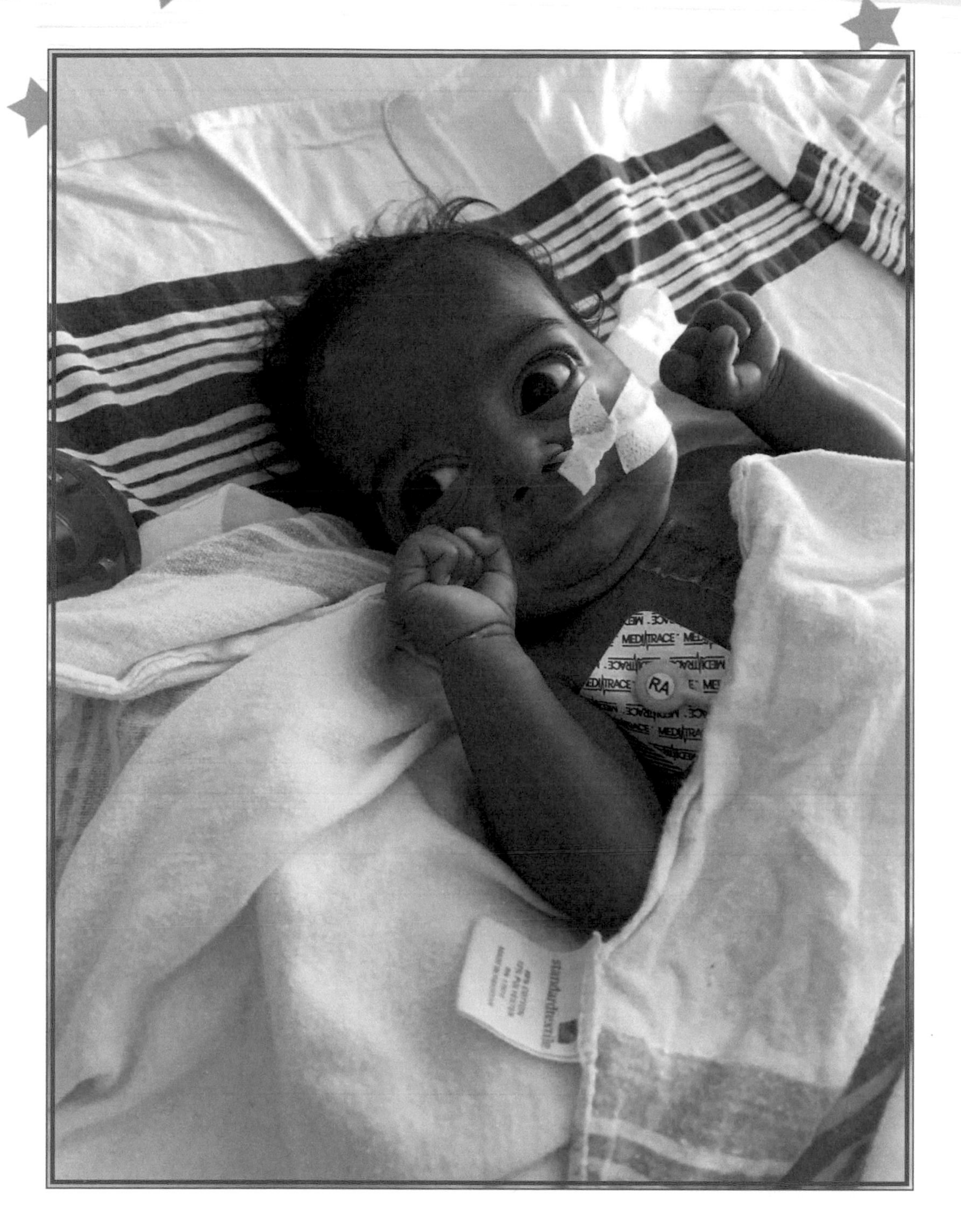

I was not able to stay the night with you the three days you were in ICU, but I was there every day to see you and called twice a day to make sure you were doing good. On Monday, February 10, 2020, you were moved back to your regular room for five more days awaiting your discharge day, which was Saturday, February 15, 2020. Mommy was so scared and excited to take you home. Before I was able to leave the hospital with you, I had to take a CPR class, a car seat class, a discharge class and training on how to place your feeding tube in your mouth and nose. The discharge class went over information how to care for you once you came home and how to administer your medication. During the discharge class I was told that babies who had heart surgery would be delayed in school. I did not accept that information and left it in God's hands. I know you will be advanced and not delayed. You came home on a feeding tube because you were still struggling with drinking out of a bottle. A week after you came home you had a home nurse who came Monday thru Friday to help me care for you.

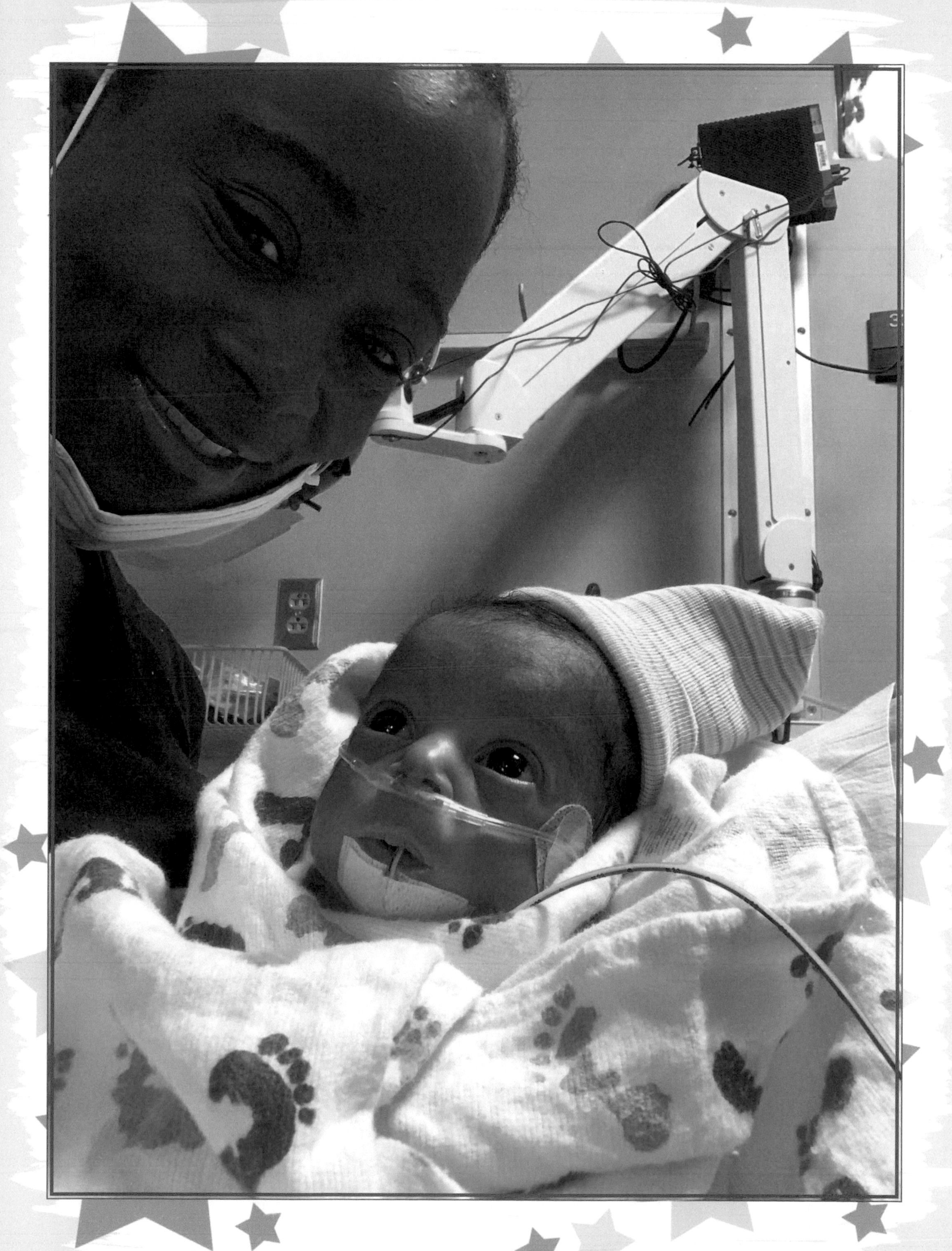

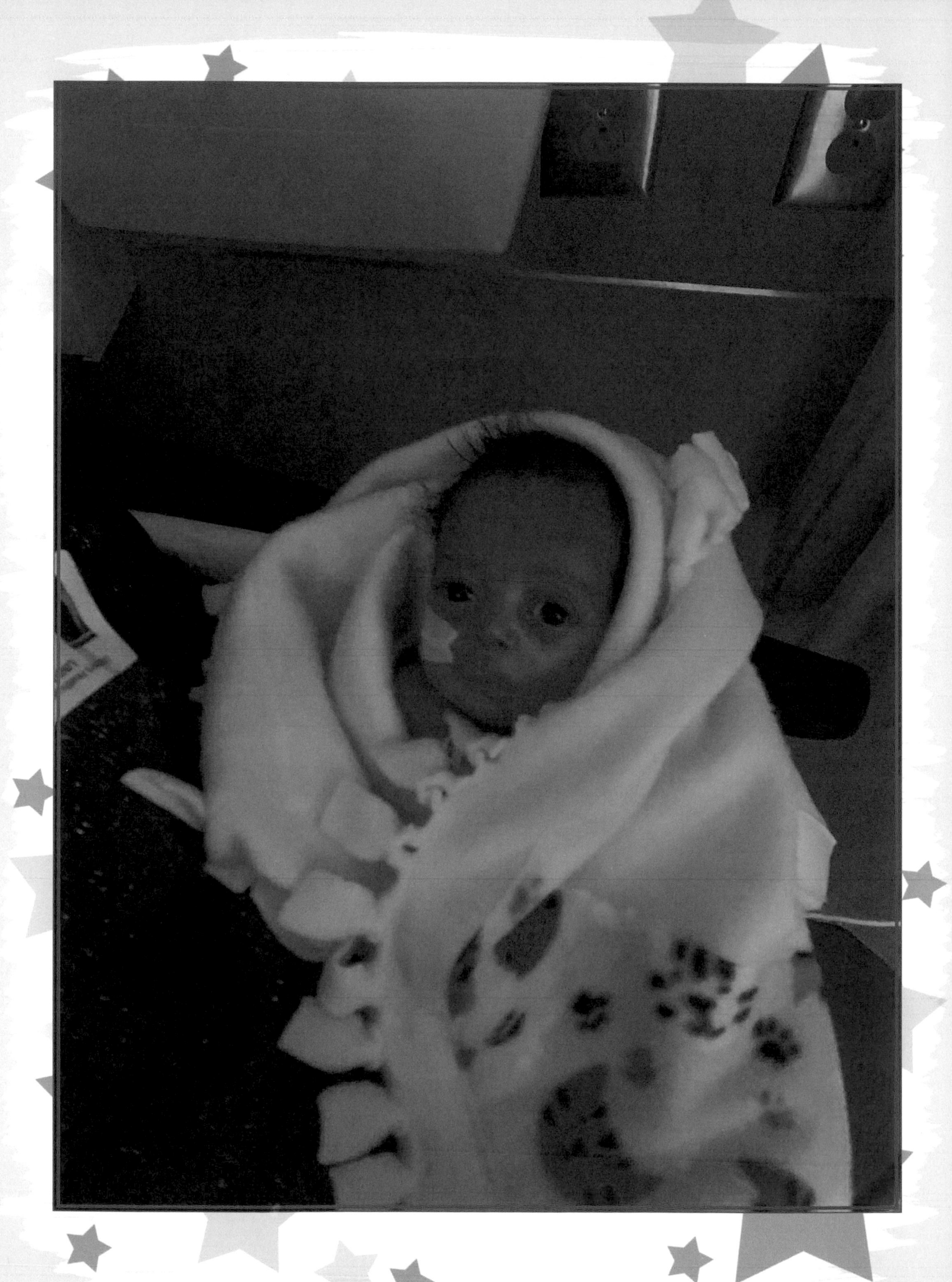

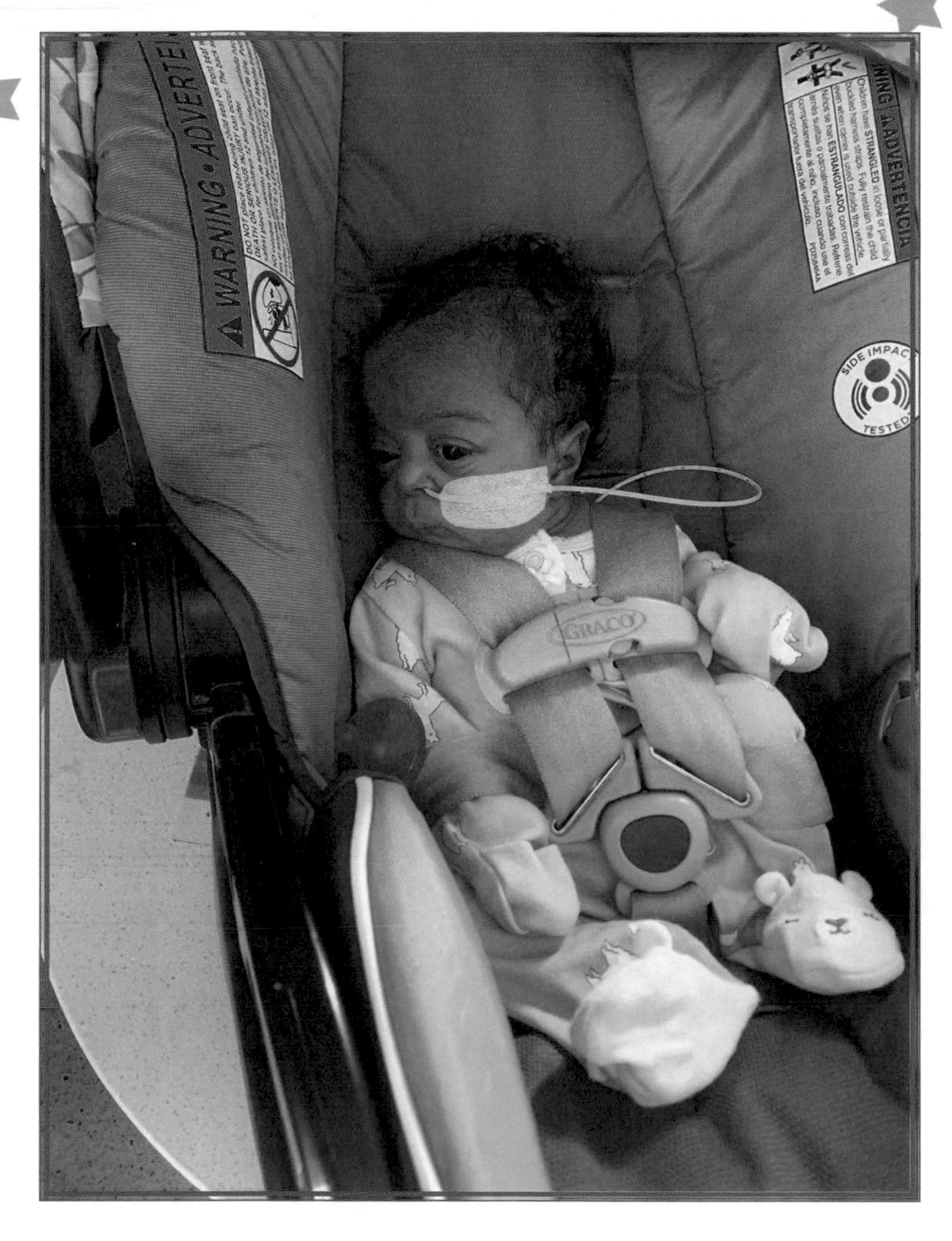

You missed major holidays like Christmas, New Years and Valentine's day. Mommy celebrated all three with you when you came home in February. You were home for St. Patrick's Day and Easter but at this time there was a worldwide pandemic in the WORLD happening called CORONAVIRUS and everyone was told to stay in their homes for weeks by President Trump. There were thousands of people who died from this virus. Your doctor appointments had to be done virtual, that means over the internet. You had a few doctors to help you through your first few months. Not only did you have your regular pediatrics to see but you had to continue to see your Cardiologist, Physical therapist and Speech pathologist. It took nine appointments to get your left ear checked. You became good friends with the Audiologist. Mommy is sharing all of this with you because I love you and hope you understand a little better the process that you had to go thru.

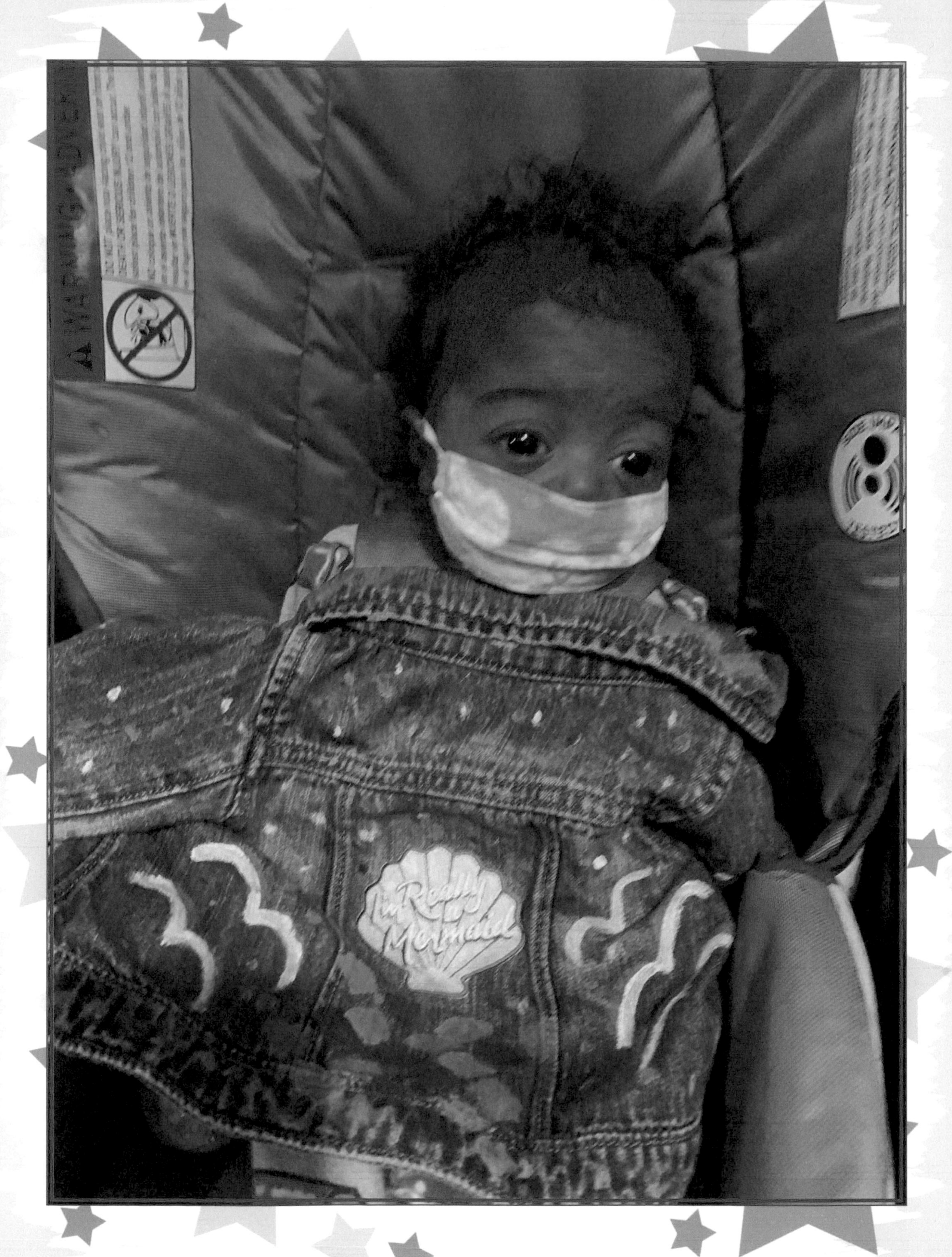
I'm Really
Mermaid

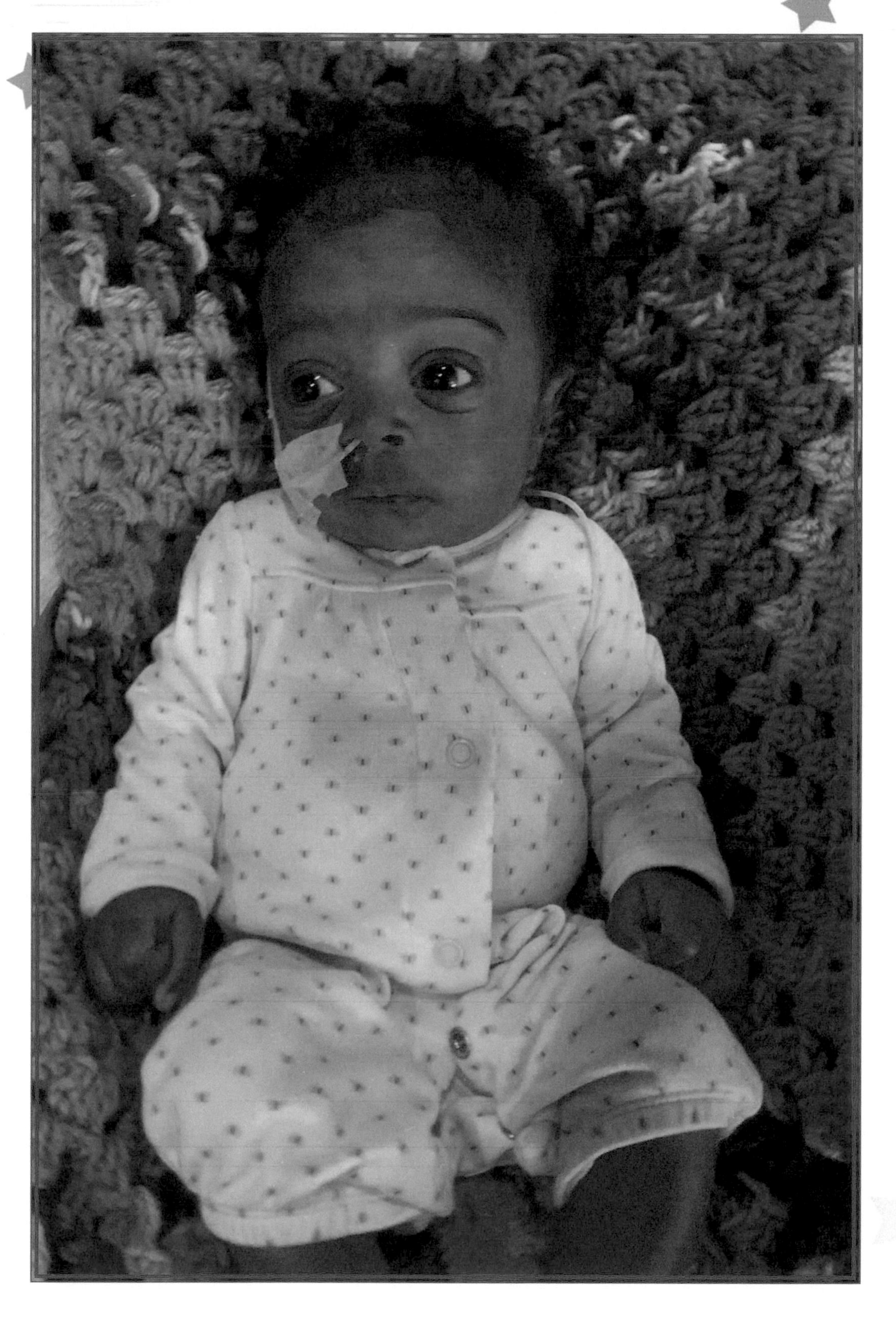

P.S. That scar on your chest is only a beauty mark from God, he also gave mommy one on her stomach where they cut you out. ***I LOVE YOU BELLA!***

Mommy…..

Printed in the United States
By Bookmasters